INTERMITTENT FASTING

*Weight Loss Guide for a Healthy Body
Burn Fat and Live a Longer Life*

ASHLEY COLLEN

Legal & Disclaimer

The information contained in this book and its contents is not designed to replace or take the place of any form of medical or professional advice; and is not meant to replace the need for independent medical, financial, legal or other professional advice or services, as may be required. The content and information in this book has been provided for educational and entertainment purposes only.

The content and information contained in this book has been compiled from sources deemed reliable, and it is accurate to the best of the Author's knowledge, information and belief. However, the Author cannot guarantee its accuracy and validity and cannot be held liable for any errors and/or omissions. Further, changes are periodically made to this book as and when needed. Where appropriate and/or necessary, you must consult a professional (including but not limited to your doctor, attorney, financial advisor or such other professional advisor) before using any of the suggested remedies, techniques, or information in this book.

Upon using the contents and information contained in this book, you agree to hold harmless the Author from and against any damages, costs, and expenses, including any legal fees potentially resulting from the application of any of the information provided by this book. This disclaimer applies to any loss, damages or injury caused by the use and application, whether directly or indirectly, of any advice or information presented, whether for breach of contract, tort, negligence, personal injury, criminal intent, or under any other cause of action.

You agree to accept all risks of using the information presented inside this book.

You agree that by continuing to read this book, where appropriate and/or necessary, you shall consult a professional (including but not limited to your doctor, attorney, or financial advisor or such other advisor as needed) before using any of the suggested remedies, techniques, or information in this book.

Table of Contents

INTRODUCTION

Whether you are trying to lose some unwanted weight or just become healthier overall, intermittent fasting should benefit you greatly. In addition to using excess cells to burn fat, and doing so at a rapid rate, intermittent fasting is incredibly fairly simple compared to other diets and does not require too many steps.

In matters of nutrition, health and weight loss, intermittent fasting has been getting quite a bit of press in the last few years. What you might not realize is that far from merely being the latest trend and brainchild of some celebrity personal trainer/nutritionist, intermittent fasting has been in existence for thousands of years! I have chosen to write this book for several reasons. First of all, I want to dispel some of the popular myths about intermittent fasting. Second, through the presentation of historical facts and the science behind fasting, I want to advocate for the efficacy of intermittent fasting. Finally, as someone who has incorporated intermittent fasting into their health regime, I want to expose you, the reader, to several variations of intermittent fasting, answer common questions people have about this health practice, offer you practical tips and tricks to get the most out of your intermittent fasting experience, help you avoid fasting mistakes and ultimately, give you the information and advice that will allow you to incorporate this health practice into your health regime as a positive life choice, that will empower you for the rest of your life!

Intermittent fasting is a process that people have been using for thousands of years for reasons ranging from spiritual to health-based. Regardless of why you are considering taking this dietary step, if you follow through with it you will see a wide variety of benefits to both your mental and your physical state.

It is not the easiest path to follow, however, especially if you are a big food fan. Luckily, the following chapters will discuss everything you need to get started practicing intermittent fasting successfully and stick with it in the long term. First you will learn all about the basics of intermittent fasting, how it works and its benefits. You will also learn about the different protocols that fall under intermittent fasting.

Read on to get more information!

CHAPTER 1

WHAT IS INTERMITTENT FASTING?

So what exactly is intermittent fasting and why does it work? Intermittent Fasting (IF) may just be the best-kept secret of the diet and fitness industry. With over 100 years of research to back up this amazing game changing lifestyle, intermittent fasting is poised to take the health and wellness community by storm.

Before we jump into what intermittent fasting is, and why it works, let's first go over a couple of things that intermittent fasting is not.

First, intermittent fasting is NOT a diet plan. There are no off-limits foods, no meal plans, no meal prepping, and no complicated recipes. In fact, you can practice intermittent fasting and eat whatever you want. You'll still get some of the benefits. Of course, intermittent fasting works the best when you try to eat more vegetables and whole foods, while eating less processed foods. It isn't necessary, and you can keep having treats without any guilt.

Second, intermittent fasting is NOT a metabolism lowering calorie restriction game. In fact, intermittent fasting can be used to lose weight, maintain weight, or even gain muscle. What does this mean for you? If you like intermittent fasting, and it ends up being a good fit, you can practice it for the rest of your life. It helps you lose weight, of course, but it has so many more benefits than just that.

Intermittent Fasting: The Basics

Let's get down to it. What is intermittent fasting? In short, intermittent fasting is a pattern of eating that involves periods of fasting, and periods of feasting. If this sounds frightening, don't worry! You've already been practicing the traditional eating pattern for your whole life.

This is what you've probably been taught: breakfast is the most important meal of the day, and you need to eat it about 30 minutes to 1 hour after you wake up. Your day should consist of three large meals, and two snacks. Many of us have been taught to believe this eating pattern is the best for our health.

But what if there was a body of research out there that proved otherwise? What if I told you that by not eating for periods of 16, 24, or even 36 hours, you could lose weight, gain muscle, and boost your energy levels and overall health? Well this is all true, and it's called intermittent fasting.

There are several different methods of intermittent fasting, and you will learn how to incorporate the top four in a later chapter. For now, let's just go over the basics. To practice intermittent fasting, you don't eat for 16+ hours. For most people, that means eating dinner at 7pm, going to sleep, and then not eating again until lunch the next day. Not eating for 16 hours might sound hard, but it becomes a lot easier if you sleep through 8 of those hours!

You may already have practiced intermittent fasting without realizing it. Have you ever woken up late on the weekend, or met a friend for a late brunch around noon? If that is your first meal of the day, you're practicing intermittent fasting.

If your first reaction to this is reluctance, keep reading. Over the next chapters, we will discuss why intermittent fasting is the right lifestyle for you and how you can easily integrate it into your life.

However, you may think to yourself, *I'll be so hungry if I skip breakfast!* We'll get more into this later, but after the first week or two, you really won't feel hungry! Your mind is used to eating in the morning, so for the first week, you will feel hungry. Once your brain learns to wait until lunch for food that hunger will go away. In many ways, intermittent fasting teaches you to listen to your body more closely.

The Science behind the Lifestyle

To convince ourselves that intermittent fasting really is the lifestyle choice for us, let's go over a few of the scientific reasons why intermittent fasting causes weight loss without damaging our metabolism.

The first truth we ought to comprehend is how the chemistry without our bodies dictates our fat loss and storage. Because when we say we want to lose weight, we mean that we want to lose fat. Now, most people follow the "calories in, calories out" method of weight loss. When you ingest fewer calories as compared to what you burn, you will lose weight. While this is true, researchers have now shown us that it leaves our metabolisms low, and we are almost guaranteed to put the weight back on.

Intermittent Fasting works because it doesn't rely on the calories in, calories out equation to promote weight loss. Instead, intermittent fasting prompts fat loss by lowering our insulin levels. So, how does insulin work?

Intermittent Fasting and Your Body's Chemistry

Insulin tells our body when it is time to store energy as fat, and when it is time to burn fat as energy. When we eat, our stomach and liver turn food into energy. Some of that energy goes into our blood stream as blood sugar, and we use that immediately. The rest? Stored as fat.

Insulin is a chemical, released by our pancreas when we eat, that tells our body it is time to store fat. So when we don't eat for 16 hours or more, our insulin level goes down significantly, and our body transitions into the fat burning mode. So, even if you ate a large dinner the night before, you'll still go into fat burning mode the next morning!

Insulin isn't the only chemical that a fast triggers, however. When we fast for longer than 16 hours, our body produces more human growth hormone (HGH). This fantastic hormone tells our body to burn fat, repair muscle, and even build new muscles! By fasting, you will lose weight and have more energy!

Yet there is even one more reason that intermittent fasting kicks the calories in calories out method of weight loss: when you fast for over 16 hours, your body produces more adrenaline. Adrenaline, in turn, gives you more energy and mental awareness! You'll feel energetic and thoughtful even when you haven't eaten recently.

The combination of these three effects, lower insulin, increased HGH, and increased adrenaline, combine in your body to raise your metabolism, sometimes up to 14% higher than your base rate. This boost in metabolism can lead to some great weight loss results! You will also be reducing your calories somewhat, since you eat fewer meals each day. This slight calorie reduction, plus increased metabolism, will lead to fantastic and long lasting results.

CHAPTER 2

HOW INTERMITTENT FASTING WORKS

Fat Burning During Fasting

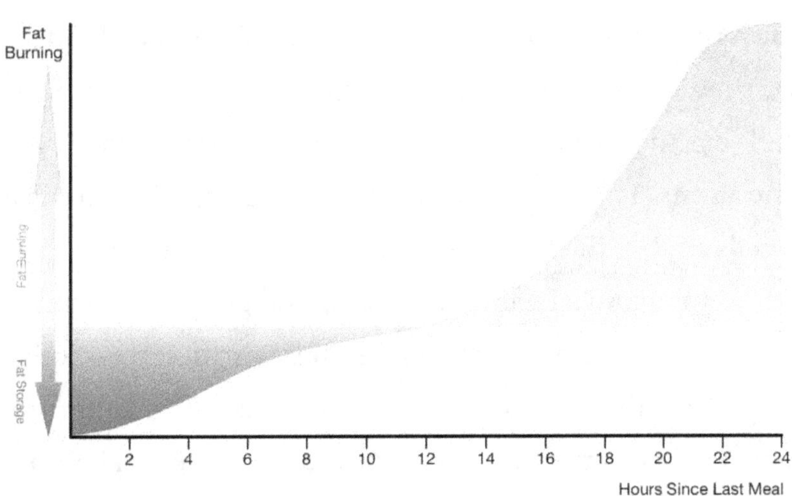

For you to understand how intermittent fasting works, it is important to understand how the body processes the food you eat.

When you eat (assuming that you follow the USDA's food pyramid, which entails high carb, minimal fat and moderate protein intake), the body goes into a fed state i.e. a state in which the body has high levels of various nutrients in the bloodstream. The fed state lasts for about 3-5 hours after which your body goes into a post-absorptive state where nothing is being digested although the levels of insulin are still high in the blood. This is the time the cells are taking up any remaining blood glucose for use or storage. During this period (the fed state and post absorptive state, the body is actively digesting everything you've eaten so that some can be absorbed into the bloodstream for transportation to different parts of the body where the cells in various parts use them for energy. After the food is absorbed and is in the bloodstream for transportation to different parts of the body, one challenge arises though; the cells don't have their own mechanism for absorbing glucose from the bloodstream. In fact, they can only do that with the aid of insulin, a hormone secreted by the pancreas in response to rising blood glucose concentrations. The purpose of insulin is simple; to 'open the gates' to the cells so that they can take up the glucose in the bloodstream in order to maintain a healthy level of blood glucose concentration. This essentially means that even if there is an excess of blood glucose (after the fed state), the presence of insulin in the bloodstream keeps the 'doors' open so that the cells take up more glucose. They don't use everything though; the excess glucose is first converted into glycogen, which is then stored in the liver. Glycogen is like an emergency/backup source of energy, which kicks in when glucose levels in the blood are low for an extended period. But the glycogen stores are limited; they can only take about 2000kcal of energy at any given time. So if there is still an excess of glucose available for the cells, it is converted into fatty acids and glycerol, which are then stored in the various fat stores around the body e.g. around organs, under the skin etc. The thing is; the presence of insulin in the bloodstream tends to promote fat storage and inhibits fat burning.

The entire process i.e. being in the fed state (up to the time the body no longer has any glucose which needs to be used up in the bloodstream) takes about 10-12 hours after you've had your meal. If you don't take any more food, this is when you start entering the fasted state, a state where the body has no more glucose in the bloodstream but is 'hungry' for nutrients. What does it do? Well, it goes to its backup power source i.e. glycogen, which it converts into glucose for use in different body processes with the help of glucagon (another hormone secreted by the pancreas) in the liver. At this time, the body doesn't just break down glycogen exclusively; it starts loosening up its grip on other energy stores e.g. the fat stores so that they can be burned to fuel different body processes. This means when you are in a fasted state (i.e. after 12-14 hours from your last meal), you can be sure of losing weight without struggle. The goal of intermittent fasting is to induce the fasted state by spacing meals in a manner that you get to a fasted state every single day so as to push your body to the point of starting to burn glycogen (and perhaps deplete it a little) so that it can start burning more stored fat for energy.

The problem with many of us is that we hardly get to the fasted state; we are very used to eating breakfast, lunch and dinner in some predetermined structure. The challenge though is that this 'structure' hardly gets us into a fasted state. In fact, we are always in the fed state, as many of us eat many meals about 4-5 hours apart. Obviously, this results in a nutrient overload and always keeps us in the fed state because this essentially keeps the body in the fed state. It is only after dinner when we try to get to the fasted state while we are asleep. But given that many of us take breakfast quite early and delay our dinner time, we hardly really 'get there'.

Do you know that this has great adverse effects on your body? Well, let me explain:

As you already know, most of the time, our bodies are in the fed state and not the fasted state making our cells more adapted to burning glucose instead of fat for energy. This simply means that normally, the levels of insulin are always high. There is a problem though; with insulin levels always high, the cells start becoming more 'dump/blind' to the signals of insulin such that more insulin is required to trigger the cells to open up to take up glucose. This is referred to as insulin resistance. In such a state, the body is always burning glucose and rarely ever burns fat (the presence of insulin has fat burning inhibitory properties) and when the glucose is depleted, the body doesn't move to the fasted stage; instead, it gets hungry for more glucose. This is because the body has less capacity to mobilize and burn fat for energy. So you can picture the cravings and the excess fat storage that comes with insulin resistance.

The secret to weight loss is in structuring your meals in a manner that ensures you get your 12-14 hours minimum from the time you had your last meal to the next. The rest of the hours i.e. 12-10 hours are really up to you; eat whatever you want but just don't overindulge! With fasting, this process goes on the reverse. When you don't eat for an extended period, the levels of insulin fall as a result of falling blood glucose levels, which signals the body to burn stored energy (glycogen and fats) since no more is coming in. This brings about weight loss in the long term.

From the above explanation, it is clear that the period within which you stay without food ought to start from about 12-14 hours (not less). If you want to fast for longer, you are free to do that; this brings about fasted effects of fasting because you get to use more of the stored fats for energy. The feeding window therefore is within 10-8 hours or less (not more).

Note: You can increase the fasting hours to achieve greater benefits. To simplify things, you can follow different intermittent fasting protocols, which we will discuss later.

So how exactly does intermittent fasting result to weight loss? Well, there are different explanations to this:

- You effectively create a calorie deficit when you fast.
- You ultimately are likely to consume fewer calories within the feeding window, something which will definitely create the much needed calorie deficit for weight loss
- You enhance your metabolism with intermittent fasting.

CHAPTER 3

BURN FAT AND LOSE WEIGHT IN A HEALTHY WAY

Most weight loss diets are complex with many rules. It is fortunate that one of the most popular fasting methods to lose weight doesn't have too many rules or conditions. Intermittent fasting keeps it simple – it is a dieting pattern where you tactically skip one or more meals for a particular period.

Intermittent fasting is not about cutting calories from your meal, but instead skipping an entire meal. This is the reason for being one of the easiest dieting patterns. The reasons behind the growing popularity of intermittent fasting are:

- Simple eating pattern

- Effectiveness to lose belly fat and reduce weight

- Other health benefits

Intermittent Fasting And Weight Loss

Intermittent fasting, as the name suggests, is a dieting pattern where you have to fast for a specific period in a day. The fasting usually lasts between 16 to 20 hours, and you eat during the other 4 to 8 hours of the day. The fasting period is referred to as the fasting window and the time you eat is known as the eating window. During the fasting window (the period you fast), you are allowed to have fluids (water, black coffee, herbal tea, etc.).

You can see better results when you spend more time fasting on a daily basis. There is no specific chart – you can fast as frequently as you prefer. The more you fast, the more effective the result.

When you follow Intermittent fasting, you gain more health benefits apart from weight loss. How does your body lose weight when you fast? Your body uses the stored body fat (nutritional reserve) for energy. This results in burning all the unwanted calories. When you burn calories in this way, you lose weight and also burn the excess fat. This will help you get a lean physique, and you will also feel healthy and energetic, as the body uses the excess body fat (stored fat) for energy. This is because it doesn't get energy from the food intake since your food intake is restricted.

Intermittent fasting helps your body to optimize the release of the major fat burning hormones – especially insulin and HGH (Human Growth Hormone) – the two most important ones. Human Growth Hormone is responsible for switching on your body's fat burning system. Your body starts to burn all the excess fat to give you the energy to carry on with your regular work (routine).

Studies show that fasting increases the production of the human growth hormone (HGH), by 2000 percent in men and 1300 percent in women.

Intermittent fasting also has a major influence on the other important hormone – insulin. It helps to keep the insulin levels steady and low, which is key to losing excess weight or avoiding extra fat from becoming accumulated in the body. Foods rich in processed carbohydrates and simple sugar accumulate more body fat. It is therefore advisable to avoid these foods as it causes the insulin levels to skyrocket and then crash whenever you eat them. This will result in excess fat accumulation in your body instead of burning it as energy.

When your insulin levels go up, you end up with health issues like obesity, Type II diabetes, and various other chronic health conditions. Intermittent fasting is the solution to all these problems. Clinical studies have proven that 15 days of consistent intermittent fasting helps to balance the insulin levels. Your body stays in a fat burning state giving you more energy all through the day.

How effective is intermittent fasting to lose fat?

Intermittent fasting encourages your body to burn more fat. Your blood sugar rises after you finish your meal. The blood sugar and the glycogen (stored carbs) in your body is the energy (your body burns), which is responsible for keeping you alive and functioning in good health. So, when you don't eat anything for a longer period, your body's blood sugar and the stored carbs go down. When it happens, your body begins to burn the stored body fat for energy.

Your body fat is nothing but the accumulation of all the excess calories that get stored in the body every time you overeat.

The body takes all these excess calories and stores them as body fat (nutritional reserve) to use as a backup energy source when:

- You become calorie-deficit due to heavy exercising or when you eat less.

- Your body is forced to burn all these excess calories, which are stored as body fat as there are not enough carbs or blood sugar to burn when you are fasting for more than 14 hours.

So, when your body fat gets burned for energy, you naturally start to lose weight as all the excess calories are getting burned.

When you combine intermittent fasting with a proper exercise plan, you tend to lose more fat and body weight thereby giving you a lean physique.

You lose fat faster when you,

- Fast for 14 to 20 hours per day

- Eat less during your weight loss diet pattern

- Combine exercising and fasting

Your metabolic rate increases when you observe intermittent fasting. This is because when your energy levels go down, along with your blood sugar levels, your body counter-reacts by releasing more adrenaline (norepinephrine). This gives you more energy and keeps you focused on your regular work routine. Since your body releases adrenaline, it forces your body to burn all the accumulated fat to provide you with energy. These stored fats are mostly found in the hips, belly and thighs.

It is true that intermittent fasting usually targets the belly fat area. It is tremendously hard to lose belly fat because the abdominal region has more alpha-2 receptors (they slow down fat burning) than the beta-2 receptors (they speed up fat burning). When you observe intermittent fasting, your insulin level goes down, which closes down the A2 receptors (as they can't work well without insulin). This will activate the B2 receptors in your abdominal region allowing your body to burn the excess fat in the belly. The increased blood flow to the belly area makes it easier for the fat-burning hormones to do their job well.

It is possible to reduce the last bit of fat your body has accumulated, through intermittent fasting. And this fasting method is essential for women as they have more fat (or A2 receptors) in their thighs, butt and hips. As mentioned earlier, the growth hormone naturally increases due to intermittent fasting and helps burn more fat. This also stops you from eating more calories as you skip one or more meals that reduce the calorie intake.

CHAPTER 4

MEDICAL BENEFITS

Intermittent fasting has helped many people lose weight and become the best versions of them. This pattern of eating is not a short-term diet, but a long-term lifestyle. Why? Because it has a whole list of research-backed health benefits that go way beyond weight loss.

Do you have complicated medical histories in your family? Maybe you're nervous about diabetes, or heart disease. The fact is, when the body is in fasting mode, you release hormones that tell the cells in your body that it is time to go into repair mode. In this repair mode, the cells can eliminate many of the first signs of disease. By practicing intermittent fasting, we give our cells more time to heal, providing ourselves with increased longevity in our lives.

Intermittent Fasting and Diabetes

The first health benefit to come from intermittent fasting originates with that little, fat regulating chemical, insulin. Insulin is probably the most famous for its role in causing or preventing the onset of diabetes.

Today, diabetes is not a debilitating disease, as long as it is caught early and dealt with responsibly. As a matter of fact, most people don't need to suffer from diabetes. Adding intermittent fasting to your lifestyle can help prevent the onset of type 2 diabetes.

Type 2 diabetes is the form of the disease that is mostly triggered by an unhealthy diet and lifestyle. The body develops insulin resistance and therefore cannot regulate the amount of sugar in the blood stream.

When we practice intermittent fasting, the body lowers its overall insulin level. Periods of low insulin help us prevent against insulin resistance. In one study conducted on human subjects, blood sugar was reduced up to 6% during a fast. During that same fast, the insulin level in the body was reduced from 20 to 31%!

A further study conducted in rats with diabetes showed that intermittent fasting helped prevent and protect the kidney from damage. This has not yet been tested in humans.

Okay, so intermittent fasting helps prevent diabetes. But what if diabetes isn't a concern for you? No one in your family has ever had diabetes and your diet right now isn't that bad. Okay, fine. What about a much more common and more deadly disease? What about cancer?

Intermittent Fasting and Cancer

It's true, intermittent fasting can help prevent and protect the body from developing certain cancers. How? Let's find out.

First, intermittent fasting has the ability to ensure that inflammation and oxidative stress in the body are reduced. *Oxidative stress* is a fancy way of talking about the cell's natural ability to detoxify itself. If this process of detoxification is interrupted or blocked, oxidative stress occurs. Unfortunately, eating a bad diet, or overeating, can lead to increased inflammation and oxidative stress in the body. These two things can lead to cancer.

There have been some studies illustrating the relationship between intermittent fasting and reduced oxidative stress and inflammation. If you're trying to prevent or even heal a chronic disease, or cancer, intermittent fasting could be an excellent choice for you.

Okay, but what if you, or someone you love, already have cancer? Based on a study done on human patients, there is some evidence that intermittent fasting can help reduce some of the side effects brought about by chemotherapy!

Probably the most important benefit of intermittent fasting is its ability to trigger autophagy in the cells. What is *autophagy*? It's a fancy way of saying "repair mode". When we are eating every three hours, cells are constantly reproducing, using the new food to create new cells. Yet when we pause and enter a short fasting period, the cells shift into repair mode.

This repair mode, known as autophagy, is essential for healthy cellular life in our bodies. Increasing the amount of repair in our bodies can protect us against certain diseases, including cancer, and Alzheimer's.

Intermittent Fasting and the Brain

Yes, that's right, IF can even help prevent Alzheimer's. The research on this claim is still rudimentary, but preliminary studies carried out on rats demonstrated that intermittent fasting can delay or slow the onset of Alzheimer's. We need more research on human studies before we can make any bolder claims than that, but for now, better safe than sorry, right?

Even if Alzheimer's isn't a concern for you, there are many more benefits to the brain from intermittent fasting. The boost that IF gives to your metabolism also impacts your brain function.

Studies in animals have revealed that intermittent fasting reduces brain damage, strokes, and improves mental functioning over time. Maybe eating your Wheaties in the morning isn't so important, after all.

Intermittent Fasting and the Heart

You may think we are done here. There can't be ANY more health benefits, right? Wrong. There is one more major health benefit to be earned from a lifestyle of intermittent fasting: lowered risk of heart disease.

Today in America, heart disease is a killer. It is one of the leading causes of death among adults, especially among adults struggling with obesity or weight gain.

Good news! Intermittent fasting has been shown, through animal studies, to improve on many different risk factors related to heart disease. It reduces blood pressure, cholesterol levels, blood triglycerides, inflammation, and blood sugar levels. Really, there can't be a better lifestyle choice out there where heart health is concerned.

Live A Longer Life

In addition to the above benefits, intermittent fasting is also known to allow those who practice it to live longer, healthier lives. Studies show that spending time in a fasting state cause your body to expend less energy on processing food, energy which is then spent on reinforcing core survival process in much the way that it does if you are starving. While your body might react to them in the same way, starving and fasting affect the body in dramatically different ways, however, which means you end up with a net positive result.

Furthermore, when your cells don't have to spend all of their time processing energy they break down more slowly which means that by practicing intermittent fasting you are ensuring that each and every part of you lives longer than it otherwise would. This, in turn, leads to an extensive range of benefits including a greatly reduced risk of cardiovascular disease and stroke. Intermittent fasting has even been proven to lessen the overall effects of chemotherapy on cancer patients. You don't need to practice intermittent fasting for a prolonged period of time to see these benefits either, they will start to manifest themselves as soon as you cut down on the number of calories you are consuming by as little as 15 percent.

CHAPTER 5

THE STYLES ON INTERMITTENT FASTING

You also need to understand everything you can about what intermittent fasting does to your body, your mind, and your life. When you understand the kind of lifestyle you are getting into and the benefits you stand to gain, then you will be able to persevere and eventually practice intermittent fasting happily and diligently. Some of the protocols you may want to look at include;

- Eat-stop-eat protocol

- The 16-8 protocol

- The 5:2 fast diet

- The alternate-day fasting

- The every-other-day protocol

16:8 Method

The 16:8 method (16 hours OFF and 8 hours ON) of Intermittent Fasting is the easiest and least hunger-inducing version of IF to integrate into your life. It is also known as the daily window fasting. This method works on its own, or as a stepping-stone towards longer fasts.

To practice 16:8 IF, you simply fast for 16 hours in a day, then eat for an 8-hour window. This is the shortest fast and the longest feasting window of any of the forms of intermittent fasting. When you follow 16:8 fasting method, you eat within the 8-hour window (maybe, 11 a.m. – 7 p.m.) and then fast for the remaining 16 hours (7 p.m. until 11 a.m.). The fasting and eating window can vary depending on the individual.

By following this form, most of your fast happens while you are asleep. It is by far the easiest style of IF for beginners. However, there are some challenges when adopting this form of intermittent fasting.

Alternate Day Fasting

If you're looking to lose a lot of weight, and you already have very strong willpower, then alternate day fasting may be the solution you have been looking for. This method can be a very extreme challenge, but if that is something you are looking for, read on.

How to Practice Alternate Day Fasting

The rules are quite simple – you fast alternate days, no calorie-intake should be present during your fast days, and you can eat normally during your eating days. Alternate Day Fasting involves not eating for a full day, every other day. Or in other words, a typical week of alternate day fasting looks like this: on Monday you don't eat, on Tuesday eat normally, on Wednesday you don't eat, on Thursday you eat normally, and so on.

Some forms of this diet allow you to eat up to 500 calories on your fasting days, but no more than that. On the non-fasting days, you can eat a normal diet. But as with any other form of intermittent fasting, it is the most effective if you commit yourself to a healthy diet rich in vegetables, fruits, and whole grains.

As with all other methods of intermittent fasting, you are allowed to drink water, black coffee, or herbal tea during your fasts, but no milk or sugar.

Eat Stop Eat

Eat Stop Eat is quickly becoming the most popular form of IF within the fasting community. Why? Because it's easy, requires little effort, saves you money, and is proven to be effective.

How to Practice Eat Stop Eat

Eat Stop Eat is quite simple, really. Eat-Stop-Eat aims to give the body a complete break from food for 24 hours. You choose two days of the week, preferably not in a row, and take a 24-hour fast. Now, the important thing to notice here is the difference between the 24-hour fast and the full day fast from the alternate day diet.

Fasting for a full day means that you don't eat at all during that day, waiting a full 36 hours before eating again. But with a 24 hour fast, the fasting window is a bit shorter. So, what would it look like in a real-life example?

On Monday, you eat normally. You have an early dinner and finish eating by 7pm. Now your fast begins. Wake up Tuesday morning and fast all day, until 7pm. At 7pm, you can have dinner. This is considerably easier, both physically and mentally, than a full 36 hour fast. You can keep your 24-hour fast from any point in the day, so breakfast to breakfast, lunch to lunch, or dinner to dinner. It doesn't matter as long as you wait the full 24 hours. And of course, water, coffee, and tea are all allowed during the fast, but no milk or sugar.

One important thing to remember is - do not exceed two fasts in one week! Fasting once in a week should be more than enough, but if you feel you can manage with two, you can still go ahead!

5:2 Diet

This style, also known as The Fast Diet, is perfect for those who are interested in trying 24 or 36-hour fasts, but who are nervous about going without food for that length of time. Though the 5:2 method of IF, you can reduce some of the stress associated with fasting by having small amounts of food during the fast.

How to Practice 5:2

The 5:2 method is a somewhat simpler method of fasting that can be used on its own, or as a stepping stone to more intense versions of intermittent fasting. So, how does this method work? You eat a normal diet for 5 days of the week, then for two days of the week you restrict your caloric intake down to 500-600 calories.

How would this work in practice? Mondays and Thursday you could eat two small meals of 300 calories or less. Every other day of the week you would eat normally. Wake up on Monday and eat a two-egg omelette with some veggies and cheese, then wait until after work and have a salad with a nice dressing. Sounds doable, right?

There shouldn't be too much of hogging or overeating on your non-fasting day – it should be the same quantity of food you eat normally. This dieting pattern is said to be the best to lose weight and improve your body's metabolic rate.

The Warrior Diet

The Warrior diet is a combination of exercise and fasting. You will need to follow your gut feeling when it comes to choosing the right diet. Avoid getting tempted by processed food or junk food. Don't get too rigid with the types of macronutrients and calories that need to be consumed during the eating window. Instead, as the name implies, eat like a warrior! Our prehistoric warriors had little food during the day and had their meal at night, i.e., little food in the day and more food at night.

The Warrior diet is more to do with vigorous exercising (even during the fasting days) and controlled food-intake. You will need to exercise when your stomach is completely empty (preferably as soon as you wake up). You will have only one meal in a day. If you can adapt to this type of intermittent fasting, you will be able to burn more fat (into energy) and will get a lean physique without the need to count your calories.

Your exercise routine should be total body strength training – squats, pushups, pull-ups, high jumps, skipping and presses. You can also include high-intensity cardio exercises, such as frog jumps or sprints, in between these sessions. These sessions can last for between 20 and 45 minutes.

Make sure you have a healthy organic, wholesome meal during your eating window. Add more vegetables, spices, greens and fruit to your plate. Drink enough water after your meal.

CONCLUSION

And with that, we have come to the end of the book. Thank you once again for choosing the book.

The book has covered the primary objective, which is to act as a beginner's guide to readers who would like to know more about intermittent fasting. The book also gives a quick overview of the role of intermittent fasting in weight loss, burning fat, maintaining a healthy body and improving lifespan.

It is essential to listen to your body and choose the fasting protocol that best suits your lifestyle, work routine and eating habits. For effective results, combine your intermittent fasting method with a good workout regimen.

I sincerely hope this book was useful and has helped in answering most of the questions you had in mind. Thanks for reading!

If you have found the information to be valuable, please write a review for the book.

Thank you!

*-- **Ashley Collen***

www.ingramcontent.com/pod-product-compliance
Lightning Source LLC
Chambersburg PA
CBHW072301260726

48658CB00002BA/939